Dedicated to

All my patients,

And my family

Amber, Ali and Sara

This book has the best dieting and antiaging techniques.

These are simple, time tested and they work.

The book is simple, straight forward and easy.

Life is beautiful

Beauty is life

You are beautiful

You are important

You are the best

Write
Your
Own
Destiny

DR J SECRETS,

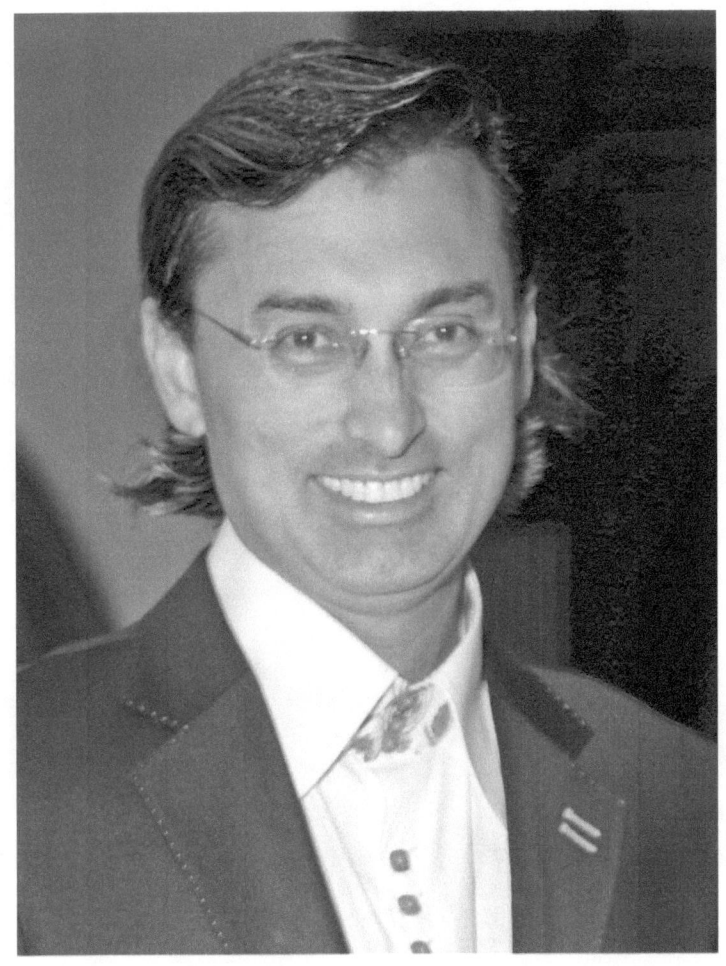

YOUNG AND SLIM FOREVER

How to be

Young and Slim

Forever !

By

Dr J

ABOUT THE AUTHOR

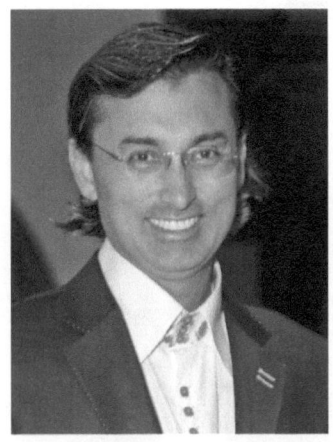

Dr. Ari-J, popularly known as **"Dr J"**, is a Board Certified Physician who has been a successful Physician and Aesthetician for many years. His main aim is to get mind, body and soul balanced. His innovative and simple methods of Dieting, The 3 G (**GGG**) approach, Weight Loss, Exercises (**Chicken trying to fly**), Anti-Aging, Relaxation, (**Balancing the Brain**), Dealing with Stress, has earned him the title of being **"Most innovative in Dieting and Weight loss."** His method of **"Avoiding Insulin Secretors"** gets a person to lose weight much faster and better than other dieting techniques. He has been on the forefront of Anti-Aging and Weight Management. Go to **DrJSecrets.com** for, Forever Beautiful, Forever Slim and Forever Young. He is sharing his many techniques and secrets in this book.

Send all inquiries to

Dr J Secrets
324 S. Beverly Drive # 403,
Beverly Hills, CA 90212
Website: www.DrJSecrets.com
Email: DrJSecrets@hotmail.com
Tel: 817-565-0922

TABLE OF CONTENTS

CHAPTER 1

AGE AND AGING

TIME AND EFFECT

What is if I tell you that there is a condition which affects more people than all the illnesses and diseases combined? This condition may be the root cause of many of the diseases themselves.

Of the longest time, mankind has been trying to answer the eternal question,

"Is there a fountain of youth?"

"Is there a fruit of longevity?"

"Is there a place where a person can live forever healthy and happy?"

Yes, you guessed it right.

The condition is Aging.

Contrary to many educated people including physicians who have tried to dodge the subject of aging saying that,

"Oh, it is just a natural process,"

I see it differently!

Time and age, maybe a natural process, but how the time affects our body, is something which can be managed and controlled.

You may have seen two brothers in the same family just a year or two apart, while one may start looking older, the other one appears young, happy and healthy. What is the difference? What is there which sets things apart?

When a person wakes up and passes the day, 24 hours pass by, is it necessary that these 24 hours produce 24 hours of age on the person, or can it be turned to only effect the aging process of an hour.

There have been many people who have tried to answer portions of the question of aging and how it affects the body, but it being a difficult subject and also not being in the main stream of medical research, these questions have not been thoroughly answered.

Does aging affect the whole person in the same way or different parts of the body differently?

You must have heard that someone went to the doctor and came back very happy saying, "My doctor said I may be 60, but I have a heart of a 20-year-old." On the other hand, somebody with back pain, who is 30 years old, have gone to a doctor and came back concerned saying that, "Oh, my doctor said, I got a spine of a 70 year-old."

Is it possible that there are specific things which can be done to slow down or halt the process of aging on those parts and overall create an effect which makes a person younger, healthier, and live a longer life?

CHAPTER 2

TIME AND NO EFFECT

I have been in medical practice for 20 years. Recently a patient said to me, "Hey Dr. J, it is good that I'm seeing you because many years ago, I used to come in to see your dad,"

I said, "it has been only me who has been the doctor here and my dad is not a physician."

He said, " 20 years ago I saw a young physician who was very nice, his name was Dr. J, and must have been your dad because you don't look old enough to be practicing that long, so you must be his son."

I said, "I remember I saw you 20 years ago and you were ill and you got better,"

The gentleman said, "Oh my God, Doc, you haven't aged a bit,"

We laughed, and I said it may be it is healthy living, good diet and exercise, or may be the good patients.

I have done things in my life which have helped me to look younger, healthier, and to the point that people would say, "Hey doc, you haven't changed much at all."

I remember going to Class Reunion and many of my friends have said, "You just look exactly the way we re-membered you.

Looking back, I wonder have I ever been sick, have I taken a sick day off.

I love taking vacations; I have traveled good, seen places, have a good family life, but not been ill.

I have been around thousands of people, many of them had medical conditions I could have had caught; infec-tions, strep, flu, stomach bugs, but I have not.

I love to listen to music, exercise, dance, go to concerts, enjoy life, also love to work on an average with more than 60 hours a week, I do all of that with a very positive attitude. Is that the reason that I still feel as young and fresh as I was when I came out of Med School. My weight is the same, energy is good.

I have been doing things which work to keep one healthy and young. I know much about aging. The balance between body, mind and soul. I know what affects these in a positive and negative way. I tell many of my patients, "be happy, be healthy, exercise, eat well, keep a good healthy weight, and follow the advice I give.

I have been practicing anti-aging and weight loss for last 20 years. Many of my patients look and feel the same as they did when they were much younger.

I have thousands of patients lose a lot of weight and they have consistently kept it off. I have combined weight loss of more than 20,000 pounds.

I have patients who have lost weight so well that their friends think they had weight loss surgery. One of my patients told me that people did not believe her that she has lost weight without surgery and she had to show her flat stomach without having a scar, for them to believe that she has not had a weight loss surgery.

I have patients who other people have asked if they did Botox or face lifts, while they have not. Their skin and face looks young and healthy. They have been following my advice and being young and healthy.

Over the years I have developed these techniques and guidelines. These work very well. These take in consideration the fast pace life now a days. These are quick, easy, do able and they work.

I have compiled these and I am putting them in the form of the book,

"Dr J Secrets. Anti-Aging and Weight Loss. How to be Young and Slim. Forever!"

CHAPTER 3

STRESS AND HOW TO DEAL WITH IT

"Nowadays, there is too much stress going on. If you switch on the TV, there is stressful news. You close the TV and turn the radio on; there is stressful news over there too.

You close the radio and try to talk to some family members, and then there is a stressful situation.

There is financial problem, there is marital problem, there is social problem, work-related issues and problems, economy, and bad news about the economy. If you go to the gas station trying to put gas in the car, dollar sign is going up and up and the gas meter is just moving a little bit.

One time I wanted to fill up gas in my car, and it stopped at $100 and the tank was still not full and no more gas to come out. I had then asked the gas attendant, he said they had put a limit on it, because they were having people drive off and not paying at times.

ALL THESE STRESSES

Stress will age you much faster. It will get you, stress you, it can even kill you. You need to be living completely stress free. Remember "Live Stress Free".

There are certain ways to deal with the stress. You can classify the stress into two different groups. One, for which you can do something about, and the other group for which you really cannot do something about.

So, you start placing your stress in the respective groups. Things you cannot do anything about, just leave them alone, there is really nothing you can do about this. Make imaginary lock boxes in your brain, put it in one of these and lock it. And throw the box and keys away.

Things you can do something about, you can classify them and see which ones are stressing you more and which ones are easily correctable. Whichever is easily correctable, get them corrected.

At least, they will not cause you anymore stress. Those which are difficult to correct, make some kind of game plan, and see what you can do to tackle them, one at a time.

Take life easy, life is too short to be stressful.

Wake up, first thing in the morning, and look yourself in the mirror and say,

"I am looking at the most handsome, beautiful, pretty and beautiful, person in the world."

"I am the most important person in the world, and I am going to take care of myself first."

With this, start your day. Do not let anything stress you out. A stress is something that will get you. It will cause you to age much faster. An hour of stress can end up putting a month of aging on your body.

You need to learn to relax. Do certain things which you know are not stressful. Which you know will relax you. Things which you want to do, like playing music, listening to music, playing a little sport, watching your favorite program, having a night out, watching a good movie, having a nice dinner for you, with your friends or significant other, boyfriend or girlfriend, husband or wife, or even with family.

Keep life in perspective. If watching TV stresses you out, watching news, especially for bad things even if they are going around the world, just turn the TV off. There is no need for you to be watching, listening, or seeing those things you really cannot do anything about, and for those things, let the people deal with them who are supposed to deal with them.

There are things at the government level, which our governments are supposed to deal with, you are not supposed to deal with them or even worry about them, or there is not even a point to even know about them.

Has watching the news and all the stressful situations going on, ever benefited you even a dime, I don't think so. Has it benefited you in the last 10, 15, 20 years, no. The only thing it has done is made you just more stressful. You need to learn to relax, don't let things bother you.

You need to cut those people off of your life, who stress you out, even if it is your family, friends or anybody else. Nobody should be giving you stress of any kind at all. If you do your work right and you do it with the fullest of your capacity and capability, that is about it. If you go to work and if somebody is stressing you out, bothering you, trying to be messy, ugly, obnoxious, you may nicely and friendly tell them not to be bad, and if they don't listen, either have them removed from the job or go get yourself another job.

You may worry about the fact that what if I leave this job, I may not be able to pay the bills or I may not get another job, don't worry about it, you are hardworking, do what you do, do it good, do it right, you will be okay.

CHAPTER 4

The following conversations "it is stressful, I'm stressed, he is stressed, she is stressed, I'm stressed out;" these have become a part of normal day conversations.

THE ANXIETY PHENOMENA

It seems that every other person who is either seeing the physicians, or at work, or in the neighborhood, or in the family, is on some kind of anti-stress, anti-anxiety medication.

At times, it seems that there is some ingredient missing from a person's daily life, which may need to just be added to the water supply or is sprayed in the air ducts to get people de-stressed or calm down.

The stress, anxiety, depression, agitation, road rage, domestic discontent, dissatisfaction at job, business, economy, all these create negative effects on the body including wrinkles on skin, headaches, reduced immunity, inability to sleep, muscle spasms, joint pains, migraines / headaches, back pain, dependence on medication, or even addiction to smoking, alcohol, or other substances creating additional negative effects on the body.

It appears that everybody is under some kind of stress. It has been shown in multiple studies that the stress and anxiety reduces longevity. Not only the reduction of age, but also appearance of being older. It increases diseases and the overall aging appearance of the person.

The fine example of this is consistently right in front of our eyes in the form of just seeing the pictures of many US presidents when they are running for election, appearing much younger than when they leave the office 4 or 8 years afterwards at which time the stress of the job has made them look much older than the actual years on the job. The term of four or eight years have made them look much older than the stated time in that term.

It appears difficult to imagine that people like the president of the United States who have access to all the resources and medical care and the help that they have, had not tried things for themselves to take care of their own aging factor and what can a common person have any more than them, which a common person can do to help them halt the process of aging. If not only halt, but may even reverse and do things which make him look much younger and healthier.

CHAPTER 5

THE DNA FACTOR

Yes, there is a natural process of a person being born and grow up to be a healthy, energetic, beautiful individual. All the information about this is stored in a person's DNA, the tiny little piece of evolutionary material which is so small that it is invisible to the naked eye; it is in fact the nucleus of every cell of human body.

It has 100s of 1000s of atoms and molecules combined in specific sequences in the form of genetic code which in simple terms can be described as looking at a railroad track in which there are two parallel tracks joined together by wooden material.

Imagine if at each wooden material interval on each side of the railroad track, there is a specific atom or a molecule, which is joined on the other side with a similar or different atom or molecule, and each of these sequenced into repetitive

2, 3, 4 or any length of different sequences; now imagine 100s of 1000s of these different sequences on these railroad tracks.

Then imagine, all these railroad tracks being taken off the ground and keeping their sequences and joints together, being rolled up into a smaller and smaller space, and then miniaturized and put into the form of DNA in every cell of the person.

Now imagine, wherever these railroad tracks have been and whatever has crossed over them, if these railroad tracks are made to remember what has happened to them, and all that information still being intact. It could be the kind of information stored, tracks from India seen the Mughal Empires and the British Forces, while tracks from France with the French revolution, while in Russia seeing Russian-speaking people, while tracks from United States with American way of life, their different stories, seasons and times.

All that information combined in one place, would be tremendous amount of data. It is out of this DNA, which certain portions are expressed to make the cell what it is in part of an organ of the body, while the other portions of this DNA dictates how this cell is going to interact with the other cells around it, and then how this organ overall is going to interact with the rest of the body.

Whenever there is an injury to the skin, the skin tends to heal, heals to a certain point when it is joined together, and then stops. Why does not it keeps on healing and keeps on just making more and more skin. These are the kind of information controlled by the DNA and the information in it.

STORAGE CAPACITY OF DNA

There have been many efforts to quantify the amount of information which is there in the human DNA and/or lab-produced DNA. In a recent research study to show the strength and the vastness of the information stored in the DNA, can you imagine what was stored as information in just one gram of DNA?

It was, 248,000 of DVDs of real time Hollywood movies which were stored in lab-made just a gram of DNA. A gram of DNA which possibly is less than the DNA of one finger that could hold 248,000 movies in it.

Not only the data of these many movies are successfully stored into the DNA, but it was transported from one point to the other and then later decoded to make those movies into the form of DVDs again. This kind of information storage capacity tells us that there is much more to learn about the actual human DNA and how it functions than just mere decoding, which was done in the Human Genome Project.

THE HUMAN GENOME PROJECT

There have been multinational efforts to decode all the sequences of the human genes and few years back, it was published as a Human Genome Project. The information is available on the internet for public, and it tells and shows where and how certain portions of the DNA are responsible for different parts of the body, including genes, which are responsible for certain diseases.

It is very exciting to see the research work of thousands of hours of hard work of great scientists, but still it makes a person wonder how does all these information relates to one own body, their own cells, longevity, and aging process.

Do the following experiment:

Take a glass of clear water, keep it static so the water is not moving, then put one drop of blue ink and watch how the blue ink still expands inside the water, initially being a drop on top of the water, the water which is apparently not moving, but quickly expanding in the form of finger-like clouds into the whole water.

Now watch as the blue ink mixes in the water and gradually the whole water turns a little blue.

Now do the same experiment again and this time take four different ink colors and put a drop of each in different portions of the top of the glass of water.

You will see each one of these inks will gradually dissipate in the same manner and at times will intertwine with the other inks and eventually will be all mixed in the water, turning the water a different color of some sort.

Did all that ink just disappear, go away, or is it still there in the water. Is it still actively interacting with the other color ink and maybe by some process each ink can be extracted back in the same original form and strength as it was put in?

Now imagine putting thousands of different color inks in the water and each one going inside the water in the same way as these few drops went in. Each one giving its own unique characteristics to the water and interacting with the water, causing the water to change, also interacting with the other inks and having the other ink interact together to make a final color. All this is an example of different pieces of evolutionary information.

This is like the human DNA making the final product, which is in the form of the human body.

CHAPTER 6

THE STRENGTH AND WEAKNESS OF HUMAN DNA

I n one regard, the human DNA is so strong, and it carries so much amount of information, it is able to express that information into the form of human being.

At the same time, there are inherent weaknesses of the DNA, especially in the form of the repair of the DNA.

This is evident in the fact that over time, with different inciting events and agents like sunlight, UV light, oxidants, free radicals, radiation, micro trauma, usage of the body organ, passage of time, portions of the DNA are constantly being weakened and broken down. There are enzymes and compounds available in the nucleus of the human cell which have to work constantly, to repair these broken down DNA.

One of the most important in the repair process is the vitamin B12. Over the years and with the advent of processed food, fast food, and the brief amount of time which people are spending in properly preparing or properly eating the meal, many of these important vitamins are either destroyed in the processing or they are not absorbed in the body.

If the DNA is not repaired correctly, the oxidants accumulate in the cells, overall reducing the health of the cell and portions of the cell, or all of the cells die, causing deterioration of the organ, in other words causing the aging process quickly. The vitamin B12 is very essential in the repair of the DNA and it not being absorbed properly in the body or not being available at the time it is needed causes gradual decline of many parts and organs of the body.

How would a person make sure that they have proper amount of vitamin B12 in their diet and it is properly absorbed in the body?

Looking into the actual science of vitamin B12 (cyanocobalamin), it is only available in food which is derived from animal products like beef, chicken, and it is not available in the plants. So, people who are purely vegetarian get weak and should take supplements of vitamin B12. Otherwise their body will get deficient in vitamin B12, eventually causing them to have reduced memory, reduced blood formation, weaknesses, nerve problems, skin problems, to the point that it has been shown that deficiency of vitamin B12 is one of the causes of having dementia and Alzheimer's disease.

It is very important to have certain amount of meat or meat products being a part of a person's diet and they should be properly eaten which means that it has to be chewed well, to be absorbed correctly; otherwise, eating a fast food burger, quickly gulping it down with a big extra-large drink, does not let the proper absorption of vitamin B12 and people get deficient in that.

The second problem is the use of antacid medications which are very widely available including medicines like Prilosec, Prevacid, Zantac, and Mylanta. These medications reduce the acid in the stomach and a certain portion of acid is necessary for the proper absorption of vitamin B12. Reduction of acid to a very low level interferes with the absorption of vitamin B12 and will cause vitamin B12 deficiency. In medical terms, the deficiency of vitamin B12 is called Pernicious Anemia.

Pernicious means very dangerous. It means not only a person's blood count will be low, but many other processes in the body will slow down.

It is also important to note that when people are healthy and young, their own body's vitamin B12 level is at a much higher level compared to when they grow older.

In many labs, the normal range of vitamin B12 is taken by doing blood test from individuals of different age group and a range is assigned, which can be anywhere from 400 to 1100 being a normal range. This is a vast and large range to be. Most of the people's own levels are at much higher when they are younger.

So, if a person who is 40 years old may do their vitamin B12 level in the blood and find out that it is 450, which may still be in the normal range, but what was it when they were 20 years old. Most probably it was in the range of 900 or a 1000. So, a level of 450 is half of what was the level for them when they were young. A reduction of 50 percent is tremendous reduction. It affects their skin tone, memory, muscle strength, and over all affects them as aging.

It is very important to have a proper nutrition, having proper vitamin B12 available in the nutrition and to give time to eat that food with small bites to chew it properly, so the vitamin B12 is absorbed in the body correctly. Also, many supplements for vitamin B12 are available including different formulations as pills, drops, multivitamin formulations, liquids, nose sprays. Many and most of these people will swallow with water not realizing that even if it's a good amount in that pill, it may not properly get absorbed until it is eaten or taken as by chewing it and swallowing it as eating a piece of food.

In my 20 years of medical practice, I have seen thousands of patients who have had multitudes of symptoms including many younger people with weakness, fatigue, tiredness, and who have gone from physician to physician and not being diagnosed and when their vitamin B12 levels are done, they are at low levels and giving them supplements or even a shot of vitamin B12 at a regimen of 1 mg given as a shot every week for eight weeks and then after, 1 mg every other week, has made a tremendous amount of improvement in their overall well-being, in their strength, stamina, in their mental alertness and focus.

I have had situations in which people have gone through medical illnesses including surgeries like a heart surgery and after the surgery had difficult recovery period and during that time, many of their weakness are rendered on being a postoperative state while when I have checked their vitamin B12 level, it had been low, and giving them a shot once a day for few days or every third day for four times, has made a tremendous difference on their ability to recover from these surgeries. Then after I had them on once a month shot and they do very well.

Because of this, I recommend every person who is 30 years or older should be taking a vitamin B12 pill and consider taking it by chewing it, not just swallowing it with water. Do the vitamin B 12 level and monitor it yearly over time. If the level at age 20 is 900, then maintain it at this level. This will keep them young and healthy for a long time. I still like the B 12 shot better, as it gets in your system much better.

After starting the B 12 therapy, the first day you will feel that your energy level is better. You are not feeling as tired as before. Same day you will feel that your memory is better. You will remember many of the things you may have forgotten, like an old password, an old friend, on old event.

The colors will feel more brighter. Vision will be crisp and thought processing will be sharper. Reflexes will be faster. Your mood will be better. Your balance will be better. Many of your aches and pains will be less.

The next day same things just more better. After few days you will feel so good and better that you may say you did not realize that you were feeling this down. Your metabolism will be better and energy level will be good and you will be able to exercise better. These are just some of the benefits of B12.

CHAPTER 7

THE DR J SKIN SECRET

———

Skin is the most important part of our body. It covers us, protects us, interacts with the outside environment at all times. It makes us beautiful and thus needs to be nurtured. It is imperative that we take the best care of our skin.

Face is the book of beauty and emotions. Being sad and worried can make you have wrinkles and lines. Being happy, smiling and laughing, exercises the good muscles of face keeping the wrinkles away.

The first and foremost is to keep skin clean. For this good mild hypoallergenic shampoo or body baths are the best choice. Skin needs to be moisturized daily. Every night take a good moisturizing lotion and rub it on the skin especially on the hands, feet, heels, between the toes and on the face. This protects them from cracking and keeps then skin healthy. Also skin is what makes you look and feel healthy and young and taking best care can have you younger looking all the time.

Over the years, I have researched and recommended specialized creams and lotions which make your skin get smooth, silky, and look much younger and healthier. These take away the wrinkles and stretch marks. Go to **DrJSecrets.com** and look for these. You will see the good effects right away. When used consistently these keeps your skin healthy, young and beautiful.

CHAPTER 8

THE DR J
HAIR SECRET

Use a mild shampoo daily and put the shampoo on the hair gently, do not rub it too much, that breaks the hair. Do not let it in too long, wash it off quickly. Let the water wash the shampoo off gently without rubbing hair. Then put a good conditioner. Conditioner can be a good strong conditioner.

Remember, it is the conditioning which keeps the hair strong and shiny. Same thing, do not rub it. Let it be in the hair for few minutes then wash it off. Let the water wash it off, without rubbing it. In this way the moisturizing and smoothing action of the conditioner will stay with the hair. Use your fingers to detangle the hair. Let it dry, using towel gently. Comb and brush gently. Do not pull hard on hair as it breaks the hair. If you break 10 hairs a day, it would mean 3000 hair gone in 300 days, don't do it. Be gentle on hair. Hair will remain healthy and shiny for long time.

Look at **DrJSsecrets.com** for more information. There are shampoo and conditioners I have used and recommend which will make the hair look and feel healthy and strong. Go to **DrJSecrets.com** to check them out.

Remember gentle shampoo, quick wash off, good conditioner, slow wash off.

CHAPTER 9

THE DR J
BONE SECRET

Taking proper care of a person's bone and joint is very important as these are the building blocks of the person's structure.

All persons should know their strength and the limit of their strength. Do not over exert the bones. Overexerting bones and joints causes joint injury and micro trauma at the surfaces of the joint. It eventually ends up causing pain and arthritis, and over a period of time they will show up as an aging process.

Taking care of a person's bones include proper rest, proper diet, proper intake of calcium and vitamin D, proper exposure to the sun to have that calcium and vitamin D converted into the active ingredients to be utilized by the bones.

It is very important to have outdoor activities with exposure to mild to moderate amount of sunlight because it is the sunlight which makes proper conversion of the vitamin D and the calcium in the body to the more useful form.

Having outdoor sports, having good walks, exercise outside on a daily basis is very important for the person's bone health. Take a good calcium and vitamin D daily. Look at **DrJSecrets.com** for further information.

CHAPTER 10

DR J
EYE SECRET

Taking care of person's eyes, as they say "eyes are the gateway to the soul" is very important. Having a proper diet including diet with vitamin A which is very essential for the health of retina, which is a back curtain of the eye on which the images are formed to be perceived by the brain.

Vitamin A is found in many vegetables including carrots and also in the form of vitamin A supplements and multivitamins. Eyes have highest number of nerves and Vitamin B 12 is very important for the nerve function. Make sure you get enough Vitamin B 12 in our diet or as a supplement.

I always recommend vitamins to be chewed and eaten as like eating a candy or a piece of food, not just being swallowing up with water. By chewing they get in the body much better.

CHAPTER 11

HORMONES

Hormones are the tiny messengers in the body which co-ordinate the care between different parts of the body.

They transmit messages from one organ to the other informing them how the other organs are functioning at an internal level.

Knowing the proper hormone balance in the body makes the body functions much better. Take for example, buying a car, putting gas in the car would be like eating the food which would make the gas in the car run, but if there is no oil, the engine would not run correctly. Similarly, if there is no grease, the wheels would not run properly.

Hormones, especially like thyroid hormone are also dependent on proper nutrition including proper amount of iodinated salts in the diet, so the thyroid gets the essential iodine it needs to make the thyroid hormone which goes and makes every part of the body work better, like the oil makes every part of the engine work better.

As a person grows older, most of the hormones levels decline. This makes person feel tired quicker and feels slower. You can get natural hormones supplements for thyroid, estrogen, and testosterone or see your physician for a one to one consultation. Remember, you do not need mega amounts of these. A smaller dose is usually ok.

Start early, have the levels checked out at younger age and keep them at same levels later, to keep looking and feeling young and healthy.

CHAPTER 12

DR J
HIGH STRESS SECRET

STRESS, HOW TO DEAL

WITH HIGH LEVELS OF IT

As there are so many stresses, what can a person do to get rid of these stresses or at least the stress not to affect them in any bad way?

There are certain things, which may stress a person out, which they can do something about and there are certain things that really cannot do anything about. So, if a person feeling stressed out, they need to think about everything, which is stressing him out and categorize it.

Put them in two categories.

Things, which you can do something about

And things, which you cannot do anything about.

Things, which you cannot do anything about, just let them alone. Forget about them because we already said we cannot do anything about them.

Thing you can do something about, you can prioritize them and see what you can do in your capacity to get something done for them and in that way, take care of one thing at a time.

DEALING WITH THE

WORLD AND STRESS

There is a lot of different things, which will stress a person out and many of them are related to person's environment including getting up, going to work, somebody stressing you out at work, your boss, your co-worker.

It may be a financial situation or a harassment situation, or family situation or friend situation. Sometimes, they all just add-up and it just becomes appearing too much. In a situation like that, going back to the basics.

Every person is born free and every person has a right to be happy.

Have confidence in yourself. When you get up in the morning, look at the mirror and say the following words.

"I am looking at the most beautiful, smart, and intelligent person in the world".

Repeat this couple of times. Make sure this gets in you really good. The next thing you say

"I am the best, I am on the top, and the rest of the people are idiots."

Now, once this fact is established say,

"Now I have to go out and face them, and let them prove to me that they are not idiots"

This means let them do something good and let me see that they are even worth worrying about. This is a very good way of dealing with too many stressful situations going on together.

Have a relaxation time, which is not involving anybody who can stress you out, any person or situation from a stressful situation. This relaxation time may be in the form of a hobby, in the form of an outing, in the form of having time for a person her or himself, and going out to eat something they like and see how that feels.

A person can find things, which they have enjoyed in the past, and because of the stressful situations, they have not been able to give time to them. List them out, one-by-one, and take time and start doing them. You will feel better.

CHAPTER 13

DR J
SLIM SECRET

OBESITY AND WEIGHT MANAGEMENT

EAT WELL, LOSE WEIGHT, FEEL GREAT, AND LIVE HEALTHY AND HAPPY

It has been a major problem for many people to control or manage their weight. Obesity and weight gain and the problems related to it have become a major issue in the United States and all across the world. It is not just a problem of the developed and Western countries, but it is an issue all over the world.

This is the way I see.

Everybody is born more or less between 6 to 8 pounds of weight.

They go through a normal upbringing with the influence of culture, place, religion and physician and medical input and it helped pretty much all over the world.

What happens between the time when they are born and when they are growing up that someone with the same amount of nutrition and culture and medical influences ends up gaining a lot more weight compared to the other people in the same situation?

Are there cultures influences, medical influences, which affect the person, with one gaining weight and becoming obese, compared to the other one, who may be normal healthy weight?

Is it a factor of how families see a child, what they want them to be, what weight they like them to be, at what point in time?

Is it the ingrained nutritional habits and instincts within the DNA and the brain of the child, which makes them eat or not eat as much, is it how their body and muscles develop, and is it the nutritional requirements of the body at different stages of life?

All of these are multifactorial influences on the person's overall weight. From the time they are born, the instincts which are ingrained in the DNA, and how they develop, how many siblings they have in the family, what is the number of the child in the sequence of the siblings, the availability of food and nutrition, and also the diseases or medical conditions which may affect the child, the availability of parental supervision and influence on the nutritional habits of the child?

All these dictate which direction the child is going to be in their weight. You may have seen two kids of the same family while they are eating the same, one may be gaining weight and one may not be.

Are there differences in their genetics, are there differences in their exercise pattern, are there any inciting events in which there are changes in the body in which how it demands nutrition and diet, how it assimilates nutrition and diet.

If the person wants to tackle their own weight, what age they are at the time they recognize and realize and want to work on having a better and healthy weight?

What social, cultural, and family support or situation that is which will help them achieve their better body weight?

The more you look into this problem, the more complex it can become and more or less out of hundreds of millions of people who are considered obese even with all the knowledge, media exposure, and medical health, only very few are ever able to effectively lose the weight and consistently keep it off.

Among all the medical, social, cultural, media jargon of obesity, why is it that obesity is still a major issue?

My approach to this is a simple approach called the **KIS, Keep It Simple**. Eat well, eat proper food, exercise well, feel great, lose weight, and keep healthy.

Food industry is the largest business for mankind and has always been, and will always be.

Food and nutrition is about the only thing which a human body consistently demands on a daily basis at least 2-3 times.

So, to keep up with this kind of demand all the businesses related to food have to compete with each other for their own survival.

Because of this, all kind of media advertisements, environment, social environment, most of religious and culture environment have pretty much one thing in common, food.

You cannot have any event, ranging from birthdays, schooling, engagements, marriage, vacations, and even to the point of funerals, they have the common element of food in them.

Whatever the ingrain, instinctual nature of the human being may be, it is influenced tremendously by the exposure to marketing material and the businesses, which are food industry related.

Ranging from domestic household food, to the fast food, to the restaurants, they all want to imprint their own stamp or the logo into the brain of the consumer.

Because of this, the instinctual nature of the nutritional demand of human body gets altered.

Depending on the environment, some families want to see their kids stronger; the others want to have their boys to excel in sports and having them healthier. Others have their multiple social gatherings in which abundant amount of high calorie foods are available.

Human body has the instinct of not just using what it needs, but also storing the extra available for any potential future needs. This instinct may be useful in the times when food supplies were inconsistent, but at this time and as in most of the countries of the world, because of the abundant food supply, this ends up accumulating more and more weight on a person.

What should be done to tackle this major problem of obesity?

What can a person do, on an individual level, on a family, social, cultural and at much bigger level, to handle this?

Can there be things which can be programed in the human brain to have it, demand and consume the amount of nutrition it needs for the healthy weight?

What can a person do on an individual level to do that?

Do we eat with our mouths and hands or the demand for food starts much before that?

There are chemical and internal hormonal changes in the body, which will initiate the demand for food.

There are clues and cues body gives which a person can tell what makes them eat more than they need.

Feeling thirsty, hungry, stressed, tired, can be these clues. Recognizing these and controlling these will help control the intake and manage the weight.

CHAPTER 14

LOSE WEIGHT, FEEL GREAT

———

To have a healthy body weight a person has to look at their daily routine and see what they can accomplish in their daily routine which will help them lose weight.

Remember, in the effort, a person's morale has to be strong, will has to be strong, and there are certain things they need to do to get this accomplished.

This is what works.

When you wake up, first thing in the morning and get out of the bed. This has to be the first thing to do. Before anything else, the first in line, not second in line. Get it to be the first in line.

Remember, first thing has to be this, The Dr J Exercise secret.

CHAPTER 15

DR J
EXERCISE SECRET

When you wake up, do this, first thing in the morning, right away. Does not matter what is going on in the world. Rain, sunshine, hot, cold weather, news, does not matter. Do not look outside window, do not see your e mail, do not turn on TV, don't look at your texts. Do a set of exercise in doing 20 slow and easy motions. This is what you do.

Stand straight, stretch your arms on the side, like an aero plane, slightly bend your knees, about 20 degrees, and keep them there, and do a bird like flying motion, with your arms moving up and down, twenty times. I call it the **"Dr. J Exercise"**, or **"Chicken trying to fly"**. After doing 20, go about your business as usual, like brush your teeth, wash your face, shower, get ready for work etc.

Now next day, do same thing but this time do thirty of these. (See Table 1, page 61). The next day do forty, and the next day, do fifty. The day after, do the first set of fifty, brush your teeth and then do another 20. Next day do the first fifty, brush your teeth, do another 30. In this way build it up to sets of 50, total ten times.

I have a 37 year old lady who is doing these and has lost from 316 to 264 pounds, that is 52 pounds in 5 months. I have another 30 year lady lost 27 pounds in 3 months. Over the years I have had combined patient weight loss of more than 20,000 pounds.

You know how long it will take you to do these, at the most 10 minutes. This is the best time investment you can do for yourself. This is one of the best exercises I have developed and it works. It makes the fat melt away and you will guaranteed lose weight. This **Dr J Chicken trying to fly**" exercise is so much fun; I have families doing it together.

It is also good for heart, brain, immune system, nerves, stress, anxiety, and overall energy. You will feel energetic the whole day. I do 500 a day. In the morning. If for any reason, I forget, I do it as soon as I can. I have even done it at the airport in the waiting lounge waiting to get on the plane. Nobody minds it. It looks like stretching. It's easy, its fun and above all it works.

I have known many people who buy treadmill, bring it home, assemble it, do it for a day or two, and then hang their towels or clothes on it. It's practically the most expansive cloth hanger there is.

The trick in exercising is doing it daily. The only way people will do it, if it is the first thing in the morning.

Life is fast, too many things to do. This exercise is quick. There are 86400 seconds in the day, this takes only maximum 600 seconds. 10 minutes out of 1440 minutes of the day. Very quick and it works. Melts the fat away. The miracle chart will get you to lose weight and inches off of your belly, for sure. You will lose 10 lb. per month.

My chicken trying to fly exercise, is so do able, I have an 80 year old lady doing 400 a day, a 74 year old blind person doing 200 a day. It's easy, it's, fun, and melts the fat away.

THE MIRACLE CHART

	X	X	X	X	X	X	X	X	X	X	
day											
1	20										
2	30										
3	40										
4	50										
5	50	20									
6	50	30									
7	50	40									
8	50	50									
9	50	50	20								
10	50	50	30								
11	50	50	40								
12	50	50	50								
13	50	50	50	20							
14	50	50	50	30							
15	50	50	50	40							
16	50	50	50	50							
17	50	50	50	50	20						
18	50	50	50	50	30						
19	50	50	50	50	40						
20	50	50	50	50	50						
21	50	50	50	50	50	20					
22	50	50	50	50	50	30					
23	50	50	50	50	50	40					
24	50	50	50	50	50	50					
25	50	50	50	50	50	50	20				
26	50	50	50	50	50	50	30				
27	50	50	50	50	50	50	40				
28	50	50	50	50	50	50	50				
29	50	50	50	50	50	50	50	20			
30	50	50	50	50	50	50	50	30			
31	50	50	50	50	50	50	50	40			
32	50	50	50	50	50	50	50	50			
33	50	50	50	50	50	50	50	50	20		
34	50	50	50	50	50	50	50	50	30		
35	50	50	50	50	50	50	50	50	40		
36	50	50	50	50	50	50	50	50	50		
37	50	50	50	50	50	50	50	50	50	20	
38	50	50	50	50	50	50	50	50	50	30	
39	50	50	50	50	50	50	50	50	50	40	
40	50	50	50	50	50	50	50	50	50	50	

Table 1, Developed By Dr J

From then on, keep on doing 10 sets of 50, every day.

I call it **THE MIRACLE CHART**. Followed daily, this is going to melt the fat away. It is simple, easy and it works. The column on the left is the day, the columns saying 20, 30, are the number of times you will do the exercise. This chart works with many exercises. The secret and the trick is doing it daily, especially first thing in the morning.

You may choose additional regime if you feel you is healthier to do it.

On the first day only do 2 jumping jacks, 2 squats, 2 sit-ups, and 2 push-ups, then next day do 3 jumping jacks, 3 squats, 3 sit-ups, 3 push-ups, then next day do 4 jumping jacks, 4 squats, 4 sit ups, 4 pushups. With this in 50 days gradually build yourself up to 50 of each. This will get your blood pumping and same way you will lose weight and inches.

I like my **Dr J Chicken trying to fly** because you can do it anywhere. You can always combine and do both in the days you can. Remember, no matter what, do the **Dr J Chicken trying to fly**, daily.

CHAPTER 16

DR J
DIET SECRET

WOW! WHAT A BREAKFAST.

ANY THING WHICH WILL NOT
HAVE YOUR BODY SECRETE
TOO MUCH INSULIN.

Everybody is different. People respond to foods differently. When a person wakes up, the body has minimal insulin levels in the blood. You want to keep it this way. Only eat the things which will not have your insulin levels increase too much.

Do the following experiment.

Try eating some food in small amount and see what happens one hour later. If it makes you much more hungry, it has caused an insulin surge in your body and for you, that food is an "insulin secretor" for you. Avoids these kinds of foods, especially in the morning.

Foods high in carbohydrate do these. Like white bread, sugar, etc. These cause an insulin surge and your glucose level drops making you much more hungry. This starts a hunger cycle and you will start eating and continue eating causing your pancreas to over work and eventually causing diabetes.

During morning time, drink one cup of hot tea. With this your body should be prepared and ready for the work ahead. Remember at this time, you do not have any insulin secretion in your body, you should not be feeling much hungry, and your body has enough reserves to start the workday.

You may want to drink a diet drink like diet coke, or coffee. Eat a light breakfast of the things which are non-insulin secretor for you. Like oat meal with skim milk is good. Avoid any sugar and sweat stuff. You may drink a diet drink like diet coke.

For me white bread is an insulin secretor. If I eat it, after an hour I feel very hungry and ends up eating more. What happens is, that it gets the insulin surge which gets the blood glucose used up and the glucose level drops.

The brain likes and survives on the glucose and wants more and makes you feel more hungry. I have a patient who cannot eat the sushi rice rolls. After eating one, he feels hungry as hell and end up eating lot more. So find the insulin secretors and avoid the insulin secretors for you.

While you are at work, at lunchtime, eat something light, especially something, which would not trigger an insulin secretion because anything heavy will have the insulin come in your system and make you feel more hungry and you will be eating more.

Things to eat at lunch would be a light salad with a little sprinkle of salt and pepper, the best salad is green vegetables, some tomatoes, and cucumber. This will keep you along good, still about 3 to 4 o'clock you may want to drink a light juice at that time. Now towards the end of the day at work, around 5 o'clock is your suppertime or dinnertime.

At that time, if you are close to home, you can wait till coming home or you can eat something at the end of your workday. The best way to eat will be to start with a salad with green vegetables, tomatoes, and red radishes. And then go to some grilled items.

TOMATOES AND RADISHES

I love the red radishes. I eat 10 of these a day. They are high in fiber. They get your stomach and intestine working good and help you absorb vitamins from food. Very very healthy for the skin and internal organs. Keeps immune system healthy and internal systems regulated.

Tomato is the best fruit of the world. Eat two a day, any kind, medium to large size. I have been eating two tomatoes a day for as long as I can remember. It is the best balanced fruit of all. It has minerals, fiber, juice, essential nutrients and very good for healthy looking skin.

Start eating 10 radishes as a salad and two tomatoes a day and within 2 days you will feel the difference in your health.

After you have had the salad, eat something like grilled chicken or grilled fish or a small piece of steak or anything you like to eat, but in smaller portion, especially make sure there is no fatty food in it.

Try to avoid cakes, regular drinks, high-sugar drinks, high or sweet stuff or too much of the sweet fruits. Remember, you can have all your minerals and vitamins, eating the fruits, which are in the vegetable category like tomatoes and peas and corn.

So you really do not have to eat sweet fruits. Sweet fruits will trigger insulin secretion and also convert into fat and increase the weight.

With these, you can go about your evening business or work with the family, with the friends, and you may want to snack a little bit at the end of the day, maybe a cookie with a small glass of milk or a salad or maybe a little piece of evening meal of some kind, which you like.

In this way, you would not feel that you have missed much of your food items and still be satisfied. Following this regimen, you will see that you will start losing weight and feeling much better.

CORN

Its everything you want it to be.

Corn is one of my favorite foods, its high in fiber, high in vitamins, and low in sugar and has no fat in it. I love eating corn and eat at least one a day. I recommend one corn boiled or microwaved for 4 minutes, to be eaten daily. It is one of the healthiest foods you can eat. Start eating one corn a day and you will feel healthy and fresh.

THE VEGETABLE OIL DRAMA

Anything, which looks like fat or oil, feels like fat, eats like fat, and if you touch it, you cannot wash it off with water only, and you have to use soap, has fat in it.

So even when the oil, say vegetable oil, corn oil, or Mazola oil, these have been chemically made and the ingredients have fat and cholesterol in it. Avoid these. These will clog your arteries.

You must have heard the plumber say, do not put greasy stuff in the drain, it clogs it up, so do not put greasy stuff in your body, it clogs it up.

THE LOW FAT LOW CHOLESTEROL LABELS

Some of the foods say low fat, low cholesterol, but you have to look at the amount of fat and amount of the cholesterol. The company may be comparing it with their own product saying low cholesterol compared to what they use to sell before.

The thing to look for is the word no cholesterol or no fat. Anything, which has no cholesterol and no fat, that thing does not have any fat or cholesterol in it and is more healthier to eat.

The word low cholesterol really does not mean anything because that food may still have a lot of fat and cholesterol in it, so that no cholesterol and no fat is the way to go.

CHAPTER 17

THE 3 G DIET (GGG)

GGG

Many people asked about the fact that how can they remember, what to eat and what not to eat and what will help them to lose weight or not gain any weight.

I call it pretty simple. It is the **GGG**, remember GGG, it stands for

G for **Green**

G for **Grilled**

G for **Good**

That mean, if it is Green, if it is Grilled, it is Good.

The first G is for Greens. Any vegetables, any food items which more or less, are green in color, especially pointing towards the green vegetables, they can be eaten in any amounts you want. They are good for digestion, good for skin, good for immune system, and good for overall health.

The second G is for grilled. You like to eat some chicken, some fish or even some beef, have it grilled.

Grilled items have all the fat melt away and you get the good protein from the food. You can combine the grilled and green that means you can have green beans, you can have salad, squash, cucumbers, or items like that, and you can even grill them with your other grilling items.

The third G is for Good. Grilled food with green vegetables is a good delicious meal.

This will help your overall body health, immune system, your strength, your muscle buildup, your stamina, so remember the **GGG**, if it is grilled, if it is green, it is good for you.

Now many people ask the question that what if they love or just would have a sweet pie, cake, chocolate, soda, wine.

I never say don't, eat any of these, you can have these, but you have to have smaller amounts of it, do not make them the large part of your meal.

THE BIRTHDAY CAKE

Everybody loves birthdays and birthday cakes. Plus like feeding you big piece of it. Take it, walk with it. Put in in file thirteen, you know what I mean. Throw it away, or put it back on the table.

By doing that and keeping this GGG acronym in your mind, you will always have the ability to remember what is good for you to eat.

You can go to a restaurant, you can go to a party, you can go to a fast food place, you can go to the grocery store and buying food for yourself, if you remember the GGG, it is green and it is grilled, it is good for you.

So remember the 3 G, GGG, and you will never falter on good and healthy foods you need to eat, to have good immune system and good skin, freshness on the face and do not gain weight and how to lose weight.

EATING OUT

All meals served in restaurants are good for two people. I always eat a salad first and then share the main course with my wife. Or get a take home box and only eat half at restaurant and bring half home to eat later. This keeps from eating any high calorie or high fat food all at once.

CHAPTER 18

DR J
BEAUTY SECRET

REMEMBER, YOU ARE BEAUTIFUL

THE BEAUTY FROM WITHIN

Can the genetic code be changed? Can the beauty from within be brought out. Can a person change how they look without expensive plastic surgery.

What you sow is what you reap. What you put in your body is what is going to show up.

Remember body is a dynamic structure and is in constant state of flux. It will respond to what you want it to be. Take an example of a butterfly. In its life cycle it goes through tremendous changes to the extent it completely transforms itself from one being to other.

From a caterpillar to a beautiful butterfly. Can similar transformation happen in a human being? Of course not to the extent of the butterfly but definitely to the extent of what a person wants to be within the confines of still being a human being.

If a person is of lighter complexion and wants the skin to appear more tan, eating foods with naturally darker pigments like black berry, brown bread, brown rice, black olives, black grapes, etc. will show up in skin darkening. At the same time getting a mild amount of sun tanning would do the trick.

Similarly getting your cheeks a rosy red color, tomatoes, red pomegranate, carrots and red radishes are very good. They will glow your cheeks red.

Wanting skin color to be lighter? Red radishes, white rice and any natural food with the inside being white will get in the body and show up under the skin and over time making it lighter. At the same time avoiding too much sunlight will definitely help in keeping skin color on the lighter side.

BEAUTY FROM OUTSIDE

Skin responds to pressure and stretch. Applied gently and consistently, skin will transform and change shape according to the desire of the person. If a person wants smaller waist size, in conjunction with diet and exercise, put an 8 inch soft binder on the abdomen. You can buy this at any exercise store or Wal-Mart, for 5 to 10 $. When put on consistently and continuously, it will reduce the size of the abdomen and bring back the stretched skin to a smaller size.

Many people have gone through weight loss surgeries and their skin ends up being loose and hanging. I recommend people going through a good counseling before they decide to have any surgery. Many people weight loss can be accomplished without the surgery. With good diet and exercise they can achieve desired weight.

At the same time having skin under mild constant pressure by a good binder type clothing and using a good anti stretch mark cream will get their skin to look lot better once weight loss is achieved and maintained.

Using a good anti-aging cream, lotion or serum on the skin will keep your skin healthy and younger looking for long. Remember the cream is usually milder, lotion is stronger and serum or plasma has the highest strength of the ingredients.

On the face there are 5 kinds of skin. Forehead, eyelids, cheeks, lips and neck. All these skins have different characteristics. They respond differently, age differently.

Creams and lotions are made for one part of the face may not work for the other part. I have recommended and used many good formulations and they work. Remember, it does not have to be strong or toxic. The trick is daily use, taking care of your skin on daily basis.

It is like you brush your teeth twice a day, shower daily, you should also take care of your skin daily. That is very important. Good cream and lotion with massaging action of your fingers increase the circulation and blood supply, makes skin healthier and younger.

Remember spend time for your skin, and do not forget the feet. Heels and toes need the same tender loving care as your face. Rub good lotion on them daily. Go to **DrJSecrets.com** for more information.

CHAPTER 19

DR J
RELAXATION SECRET

———————

Sitting position, take a deep breath in from your nose, hold it for count 3 and the breath out from the mouth pursed lip, and breath all the way out. Do it three times. It will relax your body a lot. This is a quick exercise to relax you good.

Lying down, Start from the feet, Stretch your toes five times then in your mind say " my toes are relaxing, " say this in your mind five times and feel your toes relaxing.

Then Say the same thing for your feet five times, " My feet are relaxing, ", and feel your feet relaxing, Then say the same thing for your legs, knees, thigh, hips, abdomen, chest , hands, neck face and head. This will relax your body good.

CHAPTER 20

DR J
SLEEP SECRET

———

Sleep is an essential part of the human life and an essential part of recovery process during which many organs of the body get time to recover from the use and abuse they have to suffer during the awake time.

Getting a proper sleep helps recover muscles, joints, brain, heart, even the emotions and putting the emotions in the right place is very important, and sleep plays a big part in it.

During sleep, the brain works in trying to analyze what has happened during the day and enhances the good part and suppresses the bad part. Having a good happy healthy sleep helps build healthy body and healthy emotions.

To help going to sleep, do the chapter 19 relaxation exercise, and this time, have two things additional.

Have a box fan, going on at medium speed; this makes a humming sound which masks the noises around.

Also have a soft piece of cloth rolled up and put on your eyes. I find a cotton T shirt the best for it, as it rolls up on the eyes and the sides cover the ears. It feels very comforting. It masks the light and noise. It helps getting to sleep, and staying asleep better.

Now do the above relaxation exercise and this time in your mind say the sentence, "I feel my toes going to sleep". Then say, "I feel my feet going to sleep". Keep on going up to your body and I bet as you will reach your face and eyes, you will be sleeping.

CHAPTER 21

DR J, "BALANCING THE BRAIN" SECRET

———

The human brain has two sides. They are like two drivers sitting in one car having two steering wheels. One trying to turn right and other turning left. It gets the wheels and alignment out of order, and sometimes the engine breaks down.

The sides of the brain deal with stresses differently. The left side deals with all conscience stress and right side with the subconscious stresses. The Left side memories will stress you while you are awake, while the right side will wake you up in sleep with bad dreams and you will say "Oh my God! Where did this come from?"

Buildup of the stresses in each side of the brain is like having two vertical pipes with one having too much water, with too much pressure, ready to burst, while the other having too little, at a risk of drying out.

These two sides of the brain do not connect their stresses and do not balance themselves. This even causes one sided headaches. I have developed a perfect "Balancing the Brain technique" and it works. I call it "**Dr J, Balancing the Brain Secret**"

Sit on a comfortable chair. Put both of your hands in front of you, touching the fingers and the palms, right hand touching the left, at the level of your neck. This position now connects your brain's right side to the left and left side to the right. Close your eyes. Take slow deep breaths. Feel the energy of right side flow to the left, and left side flow to the right.

Feel the thoughts of the right side flow to the left, and left side flow to the right. Let your brain loose and feel all thoughts are going away. Do this for 10 minutes or more. This will balance your brain perfectly. You will feel very refreshed and relaxed.

CHAPTER 22

REMEMBER, YOU ARE BEAUTIFUL, YOU ARE IMPORTANT, YOU ARE THE BEST.

Sleep well, wake up good, exercise every day in the morning (Chicken trying to fly), drink tea and water, take light breakfast, small lunch, eat proper supper, remember GGG, green grilled good, balance your brain, relax, do not let no one stress you, eat two tomatoes, 10 reddish, one corn, one Vitamin B 12 pill, a good multivitamin, a day.

Work well, rest well, enjoy well. You will have a young, slim, healthy and long life.

Remember, you are beautiful, you are important, you are the best.

SAMPLE DIETS MENUS

Breakfast

One tomato

One cucumber

One hot tea

One diet coke

One boiled egg

One toast

Lunch

Two tomatoes

One cucumber

One carrot

Four radishes

One piece grilled chicken or fish

Small piece of fruit

Dinner

Two tomatoes

One cucumber

One carrot

Four radishes

One piece grilled steak, fish or chicken

One small fruit

LOOK FOR
UPCOMING TITLES

Dr J Weight loss

Dr J Living without Stress

Dr J Natural Remedies

Dr J Aging to be Younger

Dr J Anti-Aging Endorsed Products

Dr J Living Worry Free, Financially

Dr J Autism, The 18 Dimensions, and How to get out, One Dimension at a time

Dr J ADHD, The truth

Dr J Relationships

Dr J Business Strategies

Dr J The I Brain

Special thanks to

All my staff

www.ingramcontent.com/pod-product-compliance
Lightning Source LLC
Chambersburg PA
CBHW020531290526
45786CB00002B/829